Notice & Disclaimer

Whilst every effort has been made by the writer and publisher to ensure the accuracy and correctness of the contents of this publication neither can be held responsible for subsequent actions taken by the reader. Even though most good quality supplements will have nothing but beneficial effects on the user it must be recognised that every individual is unique and it is possible that certain supplements could have an adverse effect when combined with mainstream pharmaceuticals for this reason qualified medical advice should always be sort from your GP or Natural Health Practitioner before starting on any course of supplements.

Contents

Vitamins

Minerals & others

Foreword

So why have we bothered to spend the time writing this book after all we get all the vitamins & minerals that we need from what we eat and drink don't we? Well that is really the point of this whole exercise, the answer is that most of us do not get all the vitamins and minerals that our bodies need for many reasons and this can be the cause of a large array of minor and major ailments. How many people have you heard complaining about not getting enough sleep, or aching badly as soon as they try and do anything of a physical nature, or lack concentration, or suffer headaches, stress, heartburn, lethargy, the list goes on and on.

Part of the problem lies in the changes to our lifestyles over the last 50 years or so, how many children do you see playing ball games in the road after school and at weekends? How many children do you see walking to school every day? How many of you have noticed that the number of cars on the road on a Sunday is now the same as the 'rush hour' of 30 years ago, this could be one of the reasons for the lack of children playing in the road, amongst other concerns. 50 years ago entertainment consisted of a little television for those who could afford one, books, cinema and clubs either sports or social that people generally walked to. Communication was face to face, telephone [landline only] or letter which took several days to get there and back again but that did not matter, it was the norm. Now from the moment that people get up they are attached to the information highway or cyberspace where everything happens instantly, the mobile phone is no longer just a telephone it is internet linked with apps for all your favourite social networks so that you do not miss out on any scrap of information. When you are not attached to your mobile phone you are in front of your work or home PC or tablet or laptop or net book connected by wifi hotspots and the like.

Now do not get me wrong I am not against change, progress or technology I am after all using a computer to prepare this book but I am concerned that the change could be far more dangerous than just a headache due to eyestrain. Many of us abuse our bodies with excessive work and the associated stresses that come with it, poor diet as a result of rushing a 'fast food' meal or worse still missing meals altogether, drinking excessive amounts of alcohol to relax or have a good time. Smoking certainly does not help but if you are a smoker you will be sick of having been told that and lack of physical exercise.

So when the first danger sign appears you rush to your GP and expect that he or she is going to wave a magic wand give you a wonder pill and all will be well again. Well be ready for the shock this is not going to happen simply because you are a highly complex organism and what's worse is that you are unique, there is not another human being the same as you so your GP is guessing at what is wrong and what is worse you will probably not be telling them the truth. The GP asks 'How many cigarettes do you smoke a day and how many units of alcohol do you drink a day?' You answer '10 and 2' because you do smoke and drink but you know your GP will give you a hard time if you tell the truth so you lie. Based on this your GP wants to encourage you to quit the evil weed and perhaps get some rest as maybe you have been over doing things a little but in reality you smoke 40 a day and drink 2 pints at lunch and 2 more in the evenings and possible 6 on Saturday and Sunday so 14 units a week becomes 52 units. What chance had your GP got of helping you?

In addition your GP has 15 minutes to identify the problem and do something about it, you are overweight, your blood pressure is a little high you are 50 years old, solution is blood test, beta blockers, aspirin & statins because the last pharmaceutical representative was very convincing concerning the latest statin that his company is making and all the field trials have proved that it is the holy grail and if he doesn't prescribe it then he is failing his patients badly. So what does he do, well he has not got the time to do all the research that he would like after all he only has 15 minutes before his next patient is sitting in front of him so he follows what the drug company's and the medical monitoring organisations tell him is best. The problem is that the pharmaceutical companies are far from impartial in the advice and information that they present to your doctor. In the same way that you are not totally honest when telling your GP how many cigarettes and how much alcohol you consume each day so it is with the pharmaceutical representative, he only passes on the information that he thinks is in his best interest in getting his drug prescribed to patients. As an example a drug company recently claimed that their Statin drug reduced heart attacks by 50% which certainly does sound very impressive particularly when you are assured that the side effects of this particular drug are no worse than for other Statin drugs. However when you look at the figures you find that in the tests carried out 3 people in 100 that had no medication suffered heart attacks compared to 2 people in a 100 who had heart attacks while taking the medication. You do not have to be a mathematician to realise that the difference is 1 in a 100 or 1% not 50% but of course 3 is 50% bigger than 2 so they have not actually lied but have instead presented the figures in a way that best serves their purpose.

But before we vilify the pharmaceutical companies we must consider that they are primarily in business to make money and the development of new drugs does involve very high development costs as well as long laboratory and field testing before there is any chance of recovering their investment. Under these circumstances is it really any wonder that they take advantage of every opportunity to promote their product whilst marginalising any negative results or side effects. So perhaps we need to keep this in mind when hearing what they are saying about their latest drug, perhaps it is not the greatest thing since sliced bread. Again I recently read a GP column in a national newspaper where the GP was commenting on the muscular pain a person was suffering by taking Statin; he commented that the benefits far outweighed the pain and lack of mobility that the patient was suffering. It appeared that the GP had become too focused on the alleged benefits of the drug and was completely ignoring the poor quality of life that was resulting from its use. What's the point of living longer if you cannot do anything without suffering severe pain?

I heard a television interview recently when a representative of the pharmaceutical industry referred to drugs as 'mainstream' and the use of herbs, vitamins and minerals as 'alternative new age' and it occurred to me that pharmaceutical medicines have only been around for about 100 years whereas the 'new age' treatments as he referred to them have been around since time began, well lets just say about 4,000 years so which would you call the alternative new age.

So, what is the alternative to the GP's course of treatment? The alternative is to prevent the problem occurring in the first place by living a more balanced life, eating a better balanced diet, supplementing with vitamins and minerals where appropriate, getting more exercise such as walking in the countryside, and restricting the things that we all know are bad for us in excess. I am not suggesting that you become a non-smoking, non-drinking, sugar free, fat free, salt free individual, many of the fads are in fact more dangerous for our health than we are led to believe.

But you have been told in the newspapers by the medical authorities and the big pharmaceutical companies that supplements are dangerous and can even kill you and that you can get all of the vitamins and minerals from the food that you eat. Okay lets just look at this for a moment, pharmaceutical companies invest vast sums of money in developing, marketing and selling drugs and their business is to make profits for their shareholders so is it possible that they have a financial interest in whether you buy vitamins or their highly priced medicine? I would not suggest, for fear of legal action, that they would lie but I think that all of us in their position would see the benefits of convincing the customer to buy our product over a competitors or an alternative. So are supplements dangerous, generally it must be said that the answer is emphatically no but there are always going to be people who are allergic to certain elements and therefore as with all things care must be taken and professional help and guidance sort. However, as an example of the scaremongering that goes on it was recently reported in the press that Vitamin C supplements in high does were dangerous and could even result in death. Even the medical profession would not put their name to this one; Vitamin C cannot be manufactured by the body and therefore has to be obtained externally, however as it is water soluble any excess is generally excreted in the urine and the sole effect is excessively yellow coloured urine. As to the risk of death, to date, worldwide the number of deaths attributed to excess consumption of Vitamin C is NIL, so where did they get their story from and what was the purpose of the story? The last part is that you can get all the vitamins and minerals from the food that you eat, well this may well have been true 50 years ago but the need to boost production has brought about the use of pesticides, fertilizers and the like which have all depleted the natural take up from the soil. In addition every plant takes a little bit of a mineral out of the soil but how does it get back into the soil, the answer is that it doesn't and therefore over a period of time the level of vitamins and minerals in the soil are reduced until next to nothing remains. We then no longer eat fresh locally grown produce; instead we buy produce that has been picked, blanched and flash frozen all of which reduces the vitamins left and available for us to eat. Worse we buy convenience foods which have been prepared for us so all that is required is 5 minutes in the microwave and they are ready to eat, the problem is the high temperatures applied to sterilise these foods also destroy the useful vitamins and minerals that did still exist in them so by the time we get to eat them most if not all the goodness has been destroyed. Finally, what do you do if you do not like the foods that contain the essential vitamin or mineral for example what do you do if you want to consume say omega 3 oil but cannot stand the taste of the fish from which it comes, mackerel, sardines, salmon and tuna are after all not to everyone's taste. Or perhaps you need vitamin C but cannot eat citrus fruits, there are alternative sources of vitamin C thankfully as it is a widely available vitamin but a supplement may be the only alternative and a deficiency of vitamin C could be a contributory factor to those winter colds that you always seem to get!!

So we need to take supplements and these can be purchased from any health food retail or online store right? Well it is correct that you can buy supplements from a wide variety of sources but are all suppliers equal? Well just like many other businesses just because they say that their products are good for you do not necessarily make it so. You see vitamins and minerals can usually be obtained from a variety of sources and some of these are easier and cheaper to use than others BUT the body does not absorb each type of the vitamin in the same way and in some cases some forms cannot be absorbed at all by the body. For example Vitamin D is fat soluble and needs to be consumed with fat to enable it to be properly absorbed and Vitamin D is necessary for the correct absorption of calcium and phosphorus which are important trace minerals. Now Vitamin D comes in two forms D-2 & D-3, D-2 is a synthetically produced version and it is what many of the cheaper supplements use, where possible the D-3 version is preferable as it is what your body uses and prefers.

In addition to the types you also need to be aware of the quantities of each vitamin or mineral contained in the product as many of the cheaper products on offer have such low levels of the active ingredients as to make them ineffective. Now the way that supplements are graded is based on the Recommended Daily Allowance or RDA which was set by governments over a period of time and in the case of some vitamins the level was set some 50 years ago. The RDA in the UK tends to be about 15% higher than that given in the US but what must be remembered is that the RDA is the minimum amount that governments believe is necessary to maintain an already healthy body and are therefore well short of those levels that are required to help a sick body heal itself. There are an alternative set of numbers named Safe Upper Limits and these are the levels that it is normally recommended to supplement to in order to heal the body. On the following pages we have given guides of the RDA for each vitamin along with some guidance as to the relative toxicity of each vitamin. However as indicated earlier the application of supplements, particularly at the higher extremes, should only occur under the close supervision of your GP or professionally qualified health advisor.

So the question that you should be asking now is "How will I know which supplements to trust?" Obviously if you have a qualified professional health advisor they should be able to guide you with this but before you put anything into your body you should be happy that you have done enough research to ensure that what you are taking is what your body needs. Below I detail 4 tips on buying supplements which have been taken from a publication by Dr John Heinerman PhD named 'Rip Off Supplements' which hopefully will be of guidance:

1. Don't buy a health supplement if its sales literature doesn't tell you **WHAT** is in it – there are a lot of fake health supplements being sold as miraculous cures for just about anything. Reputable supplement companies take great trouble to tell you exactly what's in their formulas and why.
2. Don't buy anything that doesn't tell you exactly **HOW MUCH** of a certain nutrient is present in its formula – although it may contain the correct active ingredient, if there isn't enough it won't work.
3. Don't buy a supplement if its sales literature doesn't explain **WHY** it contains certain nutrient or combination of nutrients in its formula. A common trick of dishonest supplement suppliers is to supply supplements with a long laundry list of ingredients to make them look

impressive, when in reality most of them have no reason for being there. If they don't explain why each nutrient is there, then don't buy it.

4. Get to **KNOW** the recommended daily allowances and the safe upper limits of the nutrients you want to take, so you can make an educated buying decision.

Okay now let's start looking at all the things that your body needs to remain healthy and how much of them your body needs. In the coming pages we will show you what the symptoms of a deficiency of a particular vitamin or mineral are, what are the good natural sources and detail the recommended allowances all of which you need to ensure that you make the correct decisions about your health. Towards the end we look at some other supplements as well as some commonly used herbs and finally a short list of common ailments and the generally recommended supplements to help in their treatment.

Vitamin A

Vitamin A is a fat soluble vitamin which comes in two basic forms Retinol & Beta-carotene. Retinol can be found in animal products such as eggs, butter and cod liver oil whereas Beta-carotene is found in fruits and vegetables.

Fish liver oil is the most highly recommended source for enhanced immunity however there are some drawbacks with this source that need to be kept in mind. Firstly over consumption can lead to side effects of nausea and vomiting and secondly because it is fat based the oil can become rancid if stored for a long period of time. The consumption of rancid oil can lead to disturbances of the Intestines, Liver and Spleen. It is recommended that this form of supplementation should be taken with food to aid in its absorption.

Whilst the Beta-carotene source is better as it does not suffer from the complications of rancidity or over consumption it is not a suitable source of Vitamin A for those suffering from *hyperthyroidism*. This is because those suffering from this condition lack the ability to convert the carotenoids into vitamin A and they should therefore restrict themselves to the fat based sources.

Vitamin A's importance cannot be understated as it has a significant effect on the body's immune system, skin, hair and general ability to help the body heal itself. Beta-carotene is also believed to have very strong antioxidant and anti carcinogenic properties.

It is believed that it assists in preventing the aging of the skin and is one of the reasons that many skincare products have it as an ingredient. It is also thought to improve vision and assist in preventing night blindness which is possibly where the idea that your night vision is improved by eating carrots which are of course a rich source of vitamin A. It is also believed to offer protection against glaucoma, cataracts and macular degeneration.

The symptoms of a deficiency in Vitamin A can include:
- Night Blindness
- Regular & persistent headaches
- Susceptibly to infections particularly of the chest
- Kidney Stones
- Dry and brittle hair
- Dry Eyes
- Skin problems
- Weight loss

Dosage
US RDA is 5,000 IU or 1,481mcg
EU RDA is 2,700 IU or 800mcg
SUL is 10,000 IU or 3,000mcg

As can be seen there is some variance between the recommendations from either side of the Atlantic and many health professionals do in fact recommend dosages of up to 15,000 IU for Retinol & 25,000 IU for Beta-carotene. It must be noted that Retinol is toxic and whilst 15,000 IU may be suggested it is not recommended that pregnant women take more than 5,000IU per day. Beta-carotene on the other hand is not toxic and is considered to be safe for both adults and children.

Vitamin B1

Vitamin B1 or Thiamin helps convert sugar into energy in the muscles and bones and is involved in all the key metabolic processes in the nervous system, heart, blood cells and muscles. It is found in all plant and animal foods but rich sources are whole grains, brown rice and seafood.

It has been found to be beneficial in the treatment of nervous disorders and is the only vitamin that can protect against the imbalances caused by alcoholism. There are more cases of deficiency of this vitamin than of any other and this is thought to be due to the effect of excessive alcohol consumption which in turn is believed to be related to stress.

Optimum intake of the vitamin will help us cope with stress and thereby at the same time reduce the need and desire for excessive alcohol consumption.

The symptoms of a deficiency in Vitamin B1 can include:
- Fatigue
- Irritability
- Depression
- Loss of appetite
- Muscle Weakness
- Indigestion
- Nausea

Dosage
US RDA is 1.2 – 1.5mg
EU RDA is 1.4mg
Supplements of 10-100mg

In certain circles it is recommended that the dosage be increased to between 100 – 300mg per day for heavy drinkers, smokers, pregnant women or those taking the pill. As there have been no reports of toxicity for this vitamin is believed to be safe to be consumed by all. In general cases it is suggested that it may be most beneficial as part of a daily B-complex supplement.

Vitamin B2

Vitamin B2 or Riboflavin as it is better known is a water soluble vitamin and is crucial to the production of energy and is a well known anti-oxidant. As it is water soluble it is not stored in any great amount in the body and therefore a deficiency of this vitamin can be quite common. The best natural sources of the vitamin are milk, liver, kidneys, cheese and leafy green vegetables.

It is believed that this vitamin may help protect the body against cancer, promote growth and assist in the provision of healthy skin and hair. It also helps the body metabolize fats, protein and carbohydrates, aids vision and boosts athletic performance.

The symptoms of deficiency in Vitamin B2 can include:
- Fatigue
- Reddening of the tongue
- Eczema of skin and genitals
- Cracked skin and mucus membranes

Dosage

US RDA is 1.7mg
EU RDA is 1.6mg
Supplements 10-300mg

It is suggested that an increase in intake is necessary during pregnancy, breastfeeding, taking the pill and heavy drinking. It is best taken in normal circumstances as part of a daily vitamin B complex supplement. It has been found to be toxic in very high dosages however minor rare symptoms include itching and burning of the skin.

Vitamin B3

Vitamin B3 or Niacin as it is better known is another water soluble vitamin and is essential for the synthesis of sex hormones and a healthy nervous system. Niacin is also believed to be beneficial in the treatment and prevention of schizophrenia as well as its ability to help purge toxins from the body. Natural sources of the vitamin are liver, lean meat, whole grains, peanuts, eggs and fish.

It is also believed that Niacin may assist in lowering cholesterol and thereby help maintain a healthy heart. It produces energy from sugar, fat and protein and helps to maintain healthy skin, nerves, tongue and aids digestion.

The symptoms of deficiency in Vitamin B3 can include:
- Dermatitis
- Diarrhoea
- Dementia

Dosage

US RDA is 13-18mg
EU RDA is 15-18mg
Supplements 20-100mg

Whilst large doses may be used therapeutically this should only be under the close supervision of a healthcare specialist. Indications of toxicity include depression, liver malfunction, flushing and headaches but these should only occur with doses in excess of 120mg. For general supplementation it is recommended that Vitamin B3 is taken as part of a B-complex supplement.

Vitamin B4

Adenine was at one time referred to as Vitamin B4, however it is no longer considered a true vitamin or part of the Vitamin B Complex.

Vitamin B5

Vitamin B5 otherwise known as Pantothenic Acid is another water soluble member of the B-complex family of vitamins. It is believed to help in the production of energy, helps reduce stress and controls the metabolism of fat.

This vitamin has recently gained in popularity due to the findings that suggest that not only can it boost energy levels but that it can also enhance the immune system and lower cholesterol levels and thereby help keep the heart healthy. It is also believed to encourage the healing of wounds, prevents fatigue and has been linked to the relief of arthritis.

The best natural sources include meat, whole grains, kidneys, nuts, chicken and eggs.

The symptoms of deficiency in Vitamin B5 can include:
- Fatigue
- Insomnia
- Vomiting
- Abdominal Pain

Dosage

US RDA is 10mg
EU RDA is 6mg
Supplements up to 100mg

Although there are no known toxicity issues with Vitamin B5 doses in excess of 300mg per day should only occur under the strict supervision of a healthcare professional. Once again this vitamin is best taken in general use as part of a Vitamin B-complex supplement.

Vitamin B6

Vitamin B6 is once again another of the water based vitamins that are part of the vitamin B-complex family of vitamins and is sometimes referred to as Pyridoxine. This vitamin is essential for the production of antibodies and white blood cells.

This vitamin is extremely important as it is essential for the absorption of Vitamin B12 as well as being necessary for the correct functioning of over 60 enzymes in the body. Of all the B Vitamins B6 is the most important for a healthy immune system and it is even thought to be of benefit in protecting the body from some cancers.

It is also widely used to relieve the symptoms of PMS and the menopause. In addition it is believed that this vitamin helps to control diabetes, acts as a natural diuretic and reduces muscle cramps and spasms.

The best natural sources of this vitamin are brewer's yeast, liver, kidneys, heart, melon, cabbage and eggs.

The symptoms of deficiency in Vitamin B6 can include:
- Anaemia
- Skin problems
- Nervous disorders

Dosage

US RDA is 2mg
EU RDA is 1.6-2mg
Supplements 50-200mg

This vitamin is toxic in high doses and can cause nerve damage when taken in quantities of 200mg or more a day. Should generally be taken as part of a Vitamin B-complex supplement and the use of a time release version of supplementation is considered to be the most beneficial.

Doses of more than 50mg per day should only be under the close supervision of an healthcare professional.

Vitamin B7

Biotin is not a true vitamin but because it works with B-Complex Vitamins it is often called Vitamin B7 or Vitamin H or even co-enzyme R. Biotin is water soluble and found in many foods.

The primary role of Biotin is in the metabolism of fats, proteins and carbohydrates however it is depleted by alcohol, antibiotics, cooking and refining food. Egg yolks are very high in Biotin but raw egg whites contain a protein that prevents the Biotin being absorbed.

Biotin has been linked with the prevention of hair greying and baldness. It is also believed to ease muscular aches and pains as well as treat skin conditions such as eczema and dermatitis.

Biotin works most effectively with Vitamins A, B2, B3, and B6.

Good sources of Biotin include nuts, fruits, beef, egg yolks, milk, unpolished rice and kidneys.

The symptoms of a deficiency in Vitamin B7 can include:
- Eczema
- Fatigue
- Impairment of fat metabolism

Dosage

USA RDA is 300mcg
EU RDA is 150mcg
Supplements 25 – 300mcg

Biotin is usually included in sufficient quantities in most B-Complex supplements and given the diverse range of foodstuffs that contain it obtaining sufficient may just require a slight modification of ones diet. There are no known levels of toxicity and therefore it is fairly safe to increase one's daily intake if suffering from any of the symptoms of deficiency.

Vitamin B8

Vitamin B8 otherwise known as Inositol is a water soluble fatty lipid found in many foods, was once seen as part of the B vitamin group, yet since it has been discovered to be produced by the human body from glucose, there is not sufficient evidence that shows Vitamin B8 as a vital nutrient. Some argue that it is vital to the formation of healthy cells and the triggering of calcium release in the body.

The normal benefits attributed to Vitamin B8 include a healthy immune system, nervous system and healthy skin. Similarly to Vitamin B7 it has been linked to a reduction in hair loss and may prevent greying hair. Inositol has been used effectively to treat anxiety, OCD and chronic depression. Some studies have suggested that it may also be beneficial in the treatment of patients suffering from Alzheimer's Disease and also panic disorders.

Good sources are Nuts, Beans, Seeds, Eggs, Soybeans, Legumes and Citrus Fruit.

The symptoms of a deficiency in Vitamin B8 can include:
- Loss of appetite
- Fatigue
- Dry Skin
- Nausea
- Chronic depression

Dosage

USA RDA is 40mg
EU RDA is 40mg
Supplements 100 – 3,000mg

Toxicity seems to only occur in people with already occurring disorders such as chronic renal failure and therefore there is very little risk to individuals who are not already suffering a disorder. However as always it is better to consume this compound through natural food sources if possible to decrease the likelihood of side effects or toxicity occurring.

Vitamin B9

Vitamin B9 is otherwise known as Folic Acid and is a water soluble vitamin. Everyone needs a good supply of this vitamin as it is responsible for the creation of healthy blood cells and protects them against anaemia.

There are many benefits attributed to this vitamin and one of the most notable is in the matter of human reproduction where it is essential for pregnant women to make sure that their levels are at the optimum levels as it has been shown to prevent birth defects. Other health benefits include the protection and prevention of heart disease, stroke, renal disease, cancer, obesity, depression, Parkinson's disease, schizophrenia, bone health, type 1 diabetes, macular degeneration and infertility.

Good natural sources are green leafy vegetables, whole grains, melon, avocados, yeasts,

The symptoms of a deficiency in Vitamin B9 can include:
- Weakness
- Lethargy
- Extreme Fatigue
- Sleeplessness
- Irritability
- Dementia

Dosage

US RDA is 400mcg
EU RDA is 200-360mcg
Supplements 400-800mcg

There are many people who are potentially deficient in this vitamin particularly, heavy drinkers, pregnant women, the elderly and those on a low fat diet. Given the very wide rage of foods that provide a natural source of this vitamin it should be possible to maintain normal levels by diet alone however if supplementation is required it is best taken as part of a good multivitamin and mineral supplement. This vitamin can be toxic in high doses and can cause neurological problems. Supplements of B9 should not be taken if you have or suspect a Vitamin B12 deficiency.

Vitamin B10

Also known as factor R or PABA (Para-Amino Benzoic Acid) this is a vitamin like element. Whilst it is not thought to be essential to humans it is commonly used as an additive to skincare products such as sunscreen as it is thought to lessen the risk of skin cancer. It is thought to be essential to the growth and regulation of the skin and is used to treat rheumatic fever.

In addition to the above and despite the uncertainty of its real necessity for human health it is still used as a treatment of many common ailments such as depression, eczema, irritability, fatigue, premature greying of the hair, fibrotic skin disorders and irritable bowel syndrome.

Good natural sources are leafy green vegetables, eggs, kidney, liver, mushrooms, wheat germ and whole grains.

The symptoms of deficiency in Vitamin B10 can include:
- Irritability and depression
- Constipation
- Depression
- Anxiety
- Nervousness
- Skin problems & eczema

Dosage

US RDA is 400mcg
EU RDA is 400mcg

As always it is best to try and obtain sufficient amounts of B10 from natural sources however if this is not possible and a supplementation is required then care must be taken not to consume excess amounts. The symptoms of overdose can include nausea, vomiting, skin rashes, jaundice and liver toxicity.

Vitamin B11

Vitamin B11 is another form of Folic Acid and is also known as factor S having similar properties to those of Vitamin B10.

Good natural sources are liver, heart, kidney, red meat, fish, milk, cheese and eggs.

The symptoms of deficiency in Vitamin B11 can include:
- Lack of appetite
- Weight Loss
- Nausea and vomiting
- Diarrhoea
- Fatigue

Dosage

US RDA is 200mg
EU RDA is 200mg
Supplement 100 – 3000mg

As always it is best to try and source sufficient from natural sources however if supplementation is required then high dosages should be avoided except under the supervision of a heath care professional. Can be toxic in high dosages and the symptoms of this can include nausea, vomiting, dizziness, high blood pressure, disease of the liver, kidney or heart and an increase in the requirements for magnesium and/or potassium.

Vitamin B12

Vitamin B12 otherwise known as Cobalamin is a water soluble vitamin and is once again a member of the B complex vitamin family it is also the only vitamin that contains essential minerals. This vitamin is essential for a healthy metabolism of nerve tissue and deficiencies are believed to cause brain damage and neurological disorders.

This vitamin is essential for good health and the main natural sources are liver, beef, pork, eggs, cheese and milk. In addition it is believed that vitamin B12 improves memory and concentration as well as being required to utilise fat, carbohydrates and proteins it may even be beneficial in protecting the body against cancers.

The symptoms of deficiency in vitamin B12 can include:
- Anaemia
- Mental deterioration
- Trembling

Dosage

US RDA is 6mcg
EU RDA is 5mcg
Supplements 5-50mcg

Dosages of between 5-50mcg should be adequate for most people; higher doses should be only given under the supervision of a medical professional and is best taken as part of a B-complex supplement. Vitamin B12 is not believed to be toxic.

Vitamin C

It is believed that Vitamin C is taken by more people than any other supplement however studies have shown that despite this a large percentage of the population have deficiencies. It is one of the antioxidant vitamins and is believed to boost immunity and fight cancer and infections.

Vitamin C is a water soluble vitamin which means that any excess is excreted in the urine. Its benefits include the belief that it prevents infections, assists in managing stress, speeds up healing of wounds, and helps to maintain healthy bones, teeth and sex organs. It is also believed to be an excellent natural antihistamine and that it may actually reduce the duration of colds and other viruses.

Good natural sources of Vitamin C include rosehips, blackcurrants, broccoli, citrus fruits, and all fresh fruits and vegetables.

Much of the standard Vitamin C is made from synthetic ascorbic acid which is poorly assimilated and can cause an irritation of the stomach and even lead to ulcers in extreme cases.

Non acidic sources would include Calcium Ascorbate and Ascorbyl Palmitate. Superior quality supplements would also include herbs such as fenugreek seed and marshmallow root to help protect the stomach lining and maybe ginger root or cayenne pepper to assist in its distribution throughout the body.

Citrus derived Vitamin C is preferable over the other sources as it provides a time release mechanism keeping it in the body for a longer period of time.

The symptoms of deficiency of Vitamin C can include:
- Weakness
- Poor healing ability
- Irritability
- Bleeding gums
- Loose teeth
- Bruising easily
- Joint pain

Dosage

US RDA is 60mg
EU RDA is 60mg
Supplements is up to 3,000mg

A dose of at least 60 mg a day is necessary for health but much more is required by people in at risk categories such as smokers and people suffering from stress or infection, taking antibiotics, drinking heavily or after an accident or injury. Even though vitamin C is not basically toxic it can in some people cause kidney stones and gout and with heavy doses diarrhoea and cramps. It has been suggested that it is best taken at night on an empty stomach.

Over the last 40 years there has been much discussion over what represents an acceptable intake of Vitamin C. Back in 1978 a group of eminent doctors and Nobel laureates met to discuss this very matter and the final consensus was that since vitamin C is considered a base substance that's involved in virtually all bodily functions, taking higher amounts are deemed worthwhile.

Vitamin D

Known as the sunshine vitamin this vitamin is fat soluble and can be found in most foods of animal origin. As there are no rich sources of this vitamin in food the body manufactures it in the skin from the energy of the sun. It is believed to be important for the absorption of Calcium and Phosphorus and can help to regulate Calcium metabolism.

Recent research has suggested that this vitamin may also have a role in protecting the body against some cancers and infections. Deficiency is caused by inadequate exposure to sunlight and low consumption of foods containing Vitamin D.

A very recent study has linked the re-appearance of Rickets; a disease caused by a lack of Vitamin D and thought to have been eradicated many years ago, with the increase of sun blocks. It appears that in an attempt to avoid contracting skin cancer people have followed the advice given of staying out of the sun or if out in it to cover up or use high factor sun block. The result of this preventative action has been to reduce the Vitamin D levels in the body and hence the re-appearance of Rickets.

As might be expected from the comments above Vitamin D also helps to protect against osteoporosis and is necessary for strong teeth and bones. It also along with Vitamin C boosts the immune system.

So who needs vitamin D most?
- Those living at 35°N latitude or further north. This means anyone living north of Morocco!
- Those over 50 years of age.
- Those who have dark skin.
- Those who are overweight.
- Those who are chronically ill.

The absolute best form is an oil based vitamin D preparation. Since vitamin D is fat soluble, it needs to be taken with fat in order to be properly absorbed. Vitamin D is required for the absorption and utilization of Calcium and Phosphorus.

The symptoms of a deficiency in Vitamin D can include:
- Rickets
- Osteomalacia
- Bone Pain
- Muscular weakness and spasm
- Osteoporosis
- Visual problems
- Weight loss

Dosage

US RDA is 10mcg
EU RDA is 5mcg
Supplements is 5 – 10mcg

As the best source of the vitamin is produced by the body as a result of exposure to sunlight this is perhaps the best course of action to take provided that it is done in moderation. It is estimated that an exposure of about half an hour a day should be sufficient in the UK although this may not always be possible due to the climate or time available to the individual. Natural sources that are available are oily fish such as Mackerel or in supplements such as Cod Liver Oil.

There are two common types of Vitamin D: D-3 Cholecalferol and D-2 Ergocalciferol. Avoid D-2 which is a synthetic product made by exposing certain plants to ultraviolet radiation. D-2 is not what the body naturally uses, and it falls far short in terms of efficacy. Unfortunately it just happens that many supplements are made with this version of Vitamin D. D-3 on the other hand is what your body uses and therefore prefers so try and ensure that you use this source of Vitamin D where possible, your body will thank you.

It must be born in mind that Vitamin D is the most toxic of all the vitamins and dosages should never exceed a maximum of 25mcg. Excess intake can cause nausea, vomiting, headache and depression among other symptoms. It is for this reason that the natural production by the body is perhaps the best course of action and the best medication being a stroll in the sunshine away from your desk.

Vitamin E

Is another of the fat soluble vitamins which is a key antioxidant and comes in two basic groups one is Tocopherol which is derived from saturated fats and Tocotrienols which are derived from unsaturated fats. Whilst the Tocotrienols are the most preferable since their unsaturated chain permits those to pass through denser tissue membranes more efficiently and much faster than the slower saturated versions for basic supplementation Tocopherols will do.

This vitamin has crucial antioxidant value as well as being important in the production of energy. Unlike most fat soluble vitamins Vitamin E is only stored in the body for a short time and up to 75% of its daily intake is removed from the body along with the other daily waste products.

The key role of Vitamin E is as an anticoagulant but it also has a role to play boosting the immune system and protecting against cardiovascular disease. It has also been linked with the treatment of skin problems, the prevention of miscarriage and the reduction of the symptoms of PMS.

Vitamin E naturally occurs in wheat germ, soybeans, vegetable oils, leafy green vegetables, whole grains and eggs.

There are no symptoms of a deficiency in Vitamin E.

Dosage

US RDA is 20mg
EU RDA is 18mg
Supplement is 1,000mg

It is best taken as part of a good multi vitamin and supplement preparation and although it is not generally considered to be toxic it can prove to be so with very high doses and therefore doses in excess of 600IU should only be taken under the strict supervision of a healthcare professional.

Vitamin F

When the two EFA (essential fatty acids) were discovered in 1923 they were classified as Vitamin F although subsequently they have been better classified as fats rather than vitamins. In 1934 three scientific papers were published by eminent biochemists using the name vitamin F for these unsaturated fatty acids, however in 1937 the American Medical Association completely discredited vitamin F, claiming that there was "no evidence" to justify essential fatty acids. Some 70 years later a considerable amount of scientific study has gone into confirming the importance of essential fatty acids for brain function.

Essential fatty acids are required by both humans and animals because the body requires them for good health but cannot produce them for itself. There are many different types of essential fatty acids with almost unpronounceable names such as alpha-linolenic acid – [ALA](omega 3) and linoleic acid – [LA] (omega 6).

Omega 3 fatty acids [ALA, EPA & DHA] are the most important of the Vitamin F group since they suppress inflammation which is the cause of so many of the degenerative diseases that plague us.

It is thought that insufficient EFA or the wrong balance of EFA could be a factor in a number of illnesses such as osteoporosis, heart disease, depression and also dementia.

Good natural sources of EFA are fish, shellfish, flaxseed, sunflower seeds, leafy vegetables and walnuts. For a long time Cod Liver Oil was considered an adequate source of vitamin F however when compared to Salmon, Mackerel, Herring, Anchovy and Sardines it comes up very short as Cod is predominately a low fat fish. For comparison purposes a 4 ounce piece of Salmon contains 3,600 mgs of Omega – 3 fatty acids whilst the same amount of Cod contains only 300 mgs. Of more recent years Krill has become a preferred source of Omega-3 however some of the claims made by the producers have been questioned by leading nutritional scientists. Many of the claims are based on the alleged ability of Krill oil to prevent and even reverse heart disease. The scientific evidence indicates that it is DHA that has an effect on heart disease and that this is present in all fish oil and not just in Krill. Furthermore it apparently costs more to distil DHA from Krill oil than it does from other fish oils.

Irrespective of the source any supplement should provide a predominance of EPA over DHA in the ratio of 3:1. In addition they should always be taken with food as this provides the greatest bioavailability.

There are a couple of groups that do need to beware about the consumption of Vitamin F supplements. Pregnant women should avoid plant oils such as Borage and Primrose as they have been found to on occasion induce labour. Also, Omega-6 should not be used by those who suffer epilepsy as it has been shown to induce seizures.

Finally as a curious piece of trivia it has been discovered that there is an animal that contains an alarming high level of Vitamin F in its body and it is this high level that is believed to enable it to live for so long in harsh climates. The animal can survive without food for up to a year, grow to an incredible size and live a very long life and it is the Rattlesnake! One has been recorded as being 21 feet 6 inches long, with a body of 18 inches round and an estimated age of 114 years old. So even if you live in a desert miles from any sea fish you can still get an ample supply of Vitamin F.

Vitamin K

Is a fat soluble group of Vitamins that have been found to be necessary for blood coagulation and includes two components K1 and K2. It was originally believed that a deficiency of Vitamin K was very rare unless the person was suffering from a major intestinal problem however this has since been brought into doubt as studies have found that the use of antibiotics may reduce the amount of Vitamin K in the stomach by up to 74%. Similarly diets low in Vitamin K can lead to a depletion which similarly occurs in the elderly.

In certain recent research there have been indications that vitamin K may be helpful in preventing arterial calcification which points to the possibility of it having a future role in cardiovascular disease prevention.

Natural Sources of Vitamin K are spinach, cabbage, kale, cauliflower, broccoli and Brussels sprouts. Some fruits such as avocado, kiwifruit and grapes are also high in Vitamin K.

Symptoms of a deficiency in vitamin K can include:
- Heavy menstrual bleeding
- Anaemia
- Bruising
- Nose bleeds
- Bleeding gums

Dosage

USA RDA is 90 – 120mcg
EU RDA is 120mcg
Supplement 135mg

Although there is the possibility of an allergic reaction to supplementation there is no known toxicity associated with high doses of Vitamin K. That said it is recommended that high dosages of this vitamin should only be taken under the supervision of a suitable qualified heath care professional.

Vitamin P

Vitamin P is a water soluble vitamin classified as a Bioflavonoid and as these are always associated with Vitamin C in nature they should be taken together as the former enhances the absorption of the latter. Vitamin P comes in many forms: hesperetin, hesperidin, quercetin, quercertrin, rutin and eriodictyol.

Sources include green tea and blue-green algae, supplement sources should be derived from citrus fruit peels and rose hips. The addition of bromelain, a pineapple enzyme, greatly enhances the absorption of all bioflavonoids.

As with Vitamin C, Vitamin P is best absorbed if taken at night on an empty stomach. A study undertaken in 1995 showed that the body more readily absorbs naturally occurring bioflavonoids than those that are encapsulated.

Part 2

Minerals
&
Others

Boron

Boron is a trace mineral found in plants and is essential for human health. Recent research suggests that Boron added to the diets of post-menopausal women prevented Calcium loss and bone demineralisation, a major discovery for suffers of osteoporosis. It is also claimed that in men it will raise testosterone levels and help build muscle.

Boron is found in most fruit and vegetables but is not present in meat products and therefore it is possible that meat eaters who eat a restricted fruit or vegetable diet could have a deficiency of this mineral.

A deficiency of Boron may be indicated by the following:
- Growth retardation
- Poor metabolism of Calcium, Magnesium and Phosphorus

Dosage

There are no specified figures in the US or EU for RDA but a supplement of 3mg a day is often used to prevent osteoporosis

Excessive intake of Boron can be toxic the effects of which can include a red rash, vomiting, diarrhoea, reduced circulation, shock and then coma. A fatal dose is 15 – 20g in adults and 3 – 6g in children. Symptoms start to appear at doses of above 100mg. Given the recommended daily supplement is only 3mg then these toxicity levels are substantial higher.

Calcium

Calcium is an important mineral and recent research shows that we only get about one third of what we need for good health.

It is essential for human life as it makes up bones and teeth and is crucial to enable messages to be conducted along nerves. It ensures that our muscles contract and that our hearts beat and is extremely important in the maintenance of the immune system.

There are many groups at risk of Calcium deficiency, in particular the elderly. Because it is so important to body processes our bodies take what they need from our bones which causes them to become thin and brittle.

Other than the treatment of osteoporosis Calcium has been linked with cancer prevention, the prevention of heart disease, arthritis, prevention of leg cramps and helping the body metabolise iron.

Natural sources of Calcium are dairy produce, leafy green vegetables, salmon, canned sardines and tofu.

A deficiency of Calcium may be indicated by the following:
- Rickets
- Osteoporosis
- Weak bones and teeth
- Leg cramps

Dosage

US RDA is 800 – 1,200mg
EU RDA is 800mg
Supplements 200 – 1,000mg

Experts recommend that Calcium should be taken as part of a good multi vitamin and mineral supplement although doses of up to 1,000mg may be given under the supervision of a qualified health care professional. Doses of over 2,000mg may cause hypocalcaemia but as excess Calcium is excreted it is unlikely that a toxic dose would occur.

A problem arises when it comes to using supplements to support your body's need for Calcium as this mineral comes in so many different forms and not all of them are well absorbed. The best form is Microcrystalline Hydroxyapatite Concentrate or MCHC which is derived from real bone and is very well absorbed. In addition to Calcium it also provides trace minerals of Phosphorus, Magnesium, Zinc, Copper and Iron as well as containing collagen which is the major protein found in connective tissue, cartilage and bone.

Calcium Carbonate is the principal ingredient in many Calcium supplements and can provide significant but not optimal amounts of absorbable Calcium. Because it is readily available and relatively inexpensive it is very popular although there are some concerns that it does not dissolve properly and could have a negative effect on the protection given by stomach acid against bacterial infection.

For those looking for higher calcium levels then Calcium Citrate/ Malate (CCM) is the preferred choice because of its better absorption and effectiveness in maintaining bone mass, than other Calcium supplements.

The remaining types and sources of Calcium should be avoided as whilst there is no evidence to suggest that they will harm you there is similarly no evidence that they are able to provide Calcium supplementation in the required form for the human body. They are Bone Meal, Dolomite, Calcium Stearate, Coral Calcium, Oyster Shell and D1-Calcium Phosphate.

Chromium

Chromium is a trace mineral which was discovered to be important to our health in the 1950's as it is an important regulator of blood sugar and it has been used successfully in the control and treatment of diabetes.

In addition to its role as a controller of the production of insulin it also controls the blood cholesterol levels, stimulates the synthesis of proteins and increases resistance to infection.

Good natural sources of Chromium are whole grain cereals, meat, cheese, brewers yeast, molasses and egg yolk. Fruits & vegetables have very little and refined grain products nearly none.

A deficiency in Chromium may be indicated by the following:
- Diabetes
- Nervous problems
- Heart disease
- Increased blood cholesterol levels

Dosage

There is no official Recommended Daily Allowance figure published in either the USA or EU however supplementation levels of 50 – 200mcg are normal.

As less than 10% of the mineral taken into the body is actually absorbed there is a very low risk of toxicity.

Cobalt

Cobalt is an essential trace mineral that is linked to vitamin B12 and which can assist in the prevention of anaemia. The amount in your body is dependent on how much was in the soil where your food was grown and although most people are not deficient it is more common with vegetarians.

Good natural sources of Cobalt are leafy green vegetables, meat, liver, milk, oysters and clams.

There are no specific symptoms of a deficiency of Cobalt but as previously indicated it is linked with vitamin B12 and therefore a deficiency in this vitamin is likely to lead to a deficiency in Cobalt. One symptom could be that the individual is exhibiting the signs of anaemia.

Dosage

There is no official Recommended Daily Allowance figures stated in the US or EU however the World Health Organisation recommends 1mcg.

When used therapeutically it has been found that toxicity occurred at doses over 30mg and included goitre and heart failure.

Copper

Copper is an essential trace mineral and is necessary for respiration. In conjunction with Iron, Copper is required to enable oxygen to be synthesised by red blood cells.

Copper is thought to possibly play a role in the prevention of cancer, acts as an antioxidant and boosts the immune system. It also plays a major role in the maintenance of our skin, bones and cartilage as it is required for the production of collagen.

Natural sources of Copper are animal livers, shellfish, nuts, fruit, kidneys and legumes.

Possible symptoms of a deficiency of Copper are as follows:
- Anaemia
- Oedema
- Brittle bones
- Irritability
- Loss of the sense of taste

Dosage

US RDA is 1.5 – 3mg
EU RDA is 1.2mg
Supplement is 1.5 – 3mg

Care must be taken when supplementing Copper as it can lead to a depletion of Zinc in the body however can be supplemented by means of a good quality multivitamin or by wearing a copper bracelet next to the skin.

An excess intake of Copper can cause side effects such as vomiting, diarrhoea, muscular pain and dementia however the risk of toxicity is very low.

Iron

Iron is another trace mineral which is essential for correct functioning of the human body, even the Egyptians were aware that a shortage could lead to anaemia. It is the iron present in our bodies which leads to the haemoglobin in our blood being red in colour.

Iron is required for correct muscle function and is stored in the liver, spleen, bone-marrow and muscle. It boosts energy levels and improves physical performance.

Good natural sources of Iron are shellfish, wheat bran, cereals, dried fruits, offal, brewer's yeast and cocoa powder.

Symptoms of a deficiency of Iron can include:
- Anaemia
- Tiredness
- Breathlessness
- Insomnia
- Palpitations

Dosage

USA RDA is 10 – 18mg
EU RDA is 14mg
Supplements 5 – 25mg

Pregnant and breastfeeding women, children, athletes and vegetarians may all require increased levels of iron. Supplements will be prescribed where necessary by a doctor and the normal maximum dosage is 15mg daily unless under close supervision.

Excess iron can cause constipation and diarrhoea and in extremely high doses even death although this is highly unlikely.

Magnesium

Magnesium is another mineral which is absolutely essential for the correct functioning of the human body. It is required for normal hormonal activity, the repair of cells, it also helps prevent kidney and gallstones and has proved useful in the treatment of high blood pressure.

Magnesium deficiency is very common, particularly with the elderly, heavy drinkers, pregnant women and strenuous exercisers. It has been proved that even a small deficiency can cause a disruption of the heartbeat.

Good natural sources of Magnesium are brown rice, soybeans, whole wheat flour, nuts and legumes.

Some of the symptoms of a deficiency of Magnesium are:
- Weakness
- Tiredness
- Unsteadiness
- Low blood sugar
- Palpitations
- Nervous convulsions

Dosage

US RDA is 300 – 400mg
EU RDA is 300mg
Supplements 200 – 500mg

Intake of someone eating a balanced diet is thought to be sufficient however where a deficiency is thought to exist then supplements are to be recommended. Magnesium is toxic to people suffering renal problems or atrioventricular blocks, other than these it should be considered safe.

Molybdenum

Molybdenum is an essential trace element that is a vital part of the enzyme which is responsible for the use of iron in our bodies.

It aids in the body's ability to metabolise fats and carbohydrates, helps prevent anaemia and prevents impotence.

Good natural sources of Molybdenum are wheat, wheat germ, liver, legumes, whole grains and eggs.

Symptoms of a deficiency of Molybdenum can include:
- Irregular heartbeat
- Irritability
- Inability to produce uric acid

Dosage

US RDA is 150 – 500mcg
EU RDA does not exist
Supplement 50 – 100mcg

There is still no consensus on the optimal daily intake however it is generally accepted that where there is a deficiency a supplement of between 50 – 100mcg a day is necessary to prevent ill health. Molybdenum is toxic in high doses above 10 – 15mg which can cause gout like symptoms.

Phosphorus

Phosphorus is a mineral which is essential in the body as it aids in the mineralization of the bones and teeth.

It also burns sugar for energy and acts as a co-factor for many enzymes and B – complex vitamins.

Good natural sources are yeast products, hard cheeses, canned fish, nuts, cereals and eggs.

Symptoms of a deficiency of Phosphorus can include:
- Weakness
- Bone and joint pain
- Loss of appetite
- Irritability
- Speech problems
- Mental confusion
- Anaemia
- Vulnerability to infection

Dosage

US RDA is 800 – 1,200mg
EU RDA is 800mg
Supplement 1,000mg

A deficiency in Phosphorous is usually accompanied with a deficiency of Potassium, Magnesium and Zinc and therefore treatment is by far best dealt with by the use of a good multivitamin and mineral supplement. Toxicity may occur with dosages over 1,000mg a day and may cause diarrhoea, calcification of organs and the prevention of the absorption of certain other minerals.

Potassium

Potassium is one of the most important minerals in our bodies. It not only links with other minerals such as Sodium to form the electrolytes which make up our bodily fluids but is also essential for the correct functioning of our nervous system, heartbeat, energy production and muscle function.

It helps to maintain the correct water balance in the cells of the body and stabilise their internal structure, helps with athletic performance and may assist in preventing cancer.

Good natural sources of Potassium are fresh fruit and vegetables and in particular bananas, melons, raisins and dried apricots and prunes since they are all high in naturally occurring Potassium Citrate.

Symptoms of a deficiency of Potassium may include:
- Vomiting
- Muscle pains
- Fatigue
- Irregular heartbeat
- Low blood pressure

Dosage

US RDA is 900mg
EU RDA is 3,500mg

Potassium is rarely given as a supplement although it is sometimes prescribed and administered under strict medical supervision. There are five usable forms of Potassium and of these Potassium Chloride is the preferred version of the medical profession due to the fact that it raises the blood levels of Potassium faster than any of the other forms. But as indicated above this is only administered under strict medical supervision. Supplement manufacturers often use small amounts of both Potassium Chloride and Potassium Citrate in their mineral products. The problem with Potassium Citrate in such supplements is that it can dramatically increase personal Potassium levels if taken for very long.

While supplements are important and hold their rightful place in optimal nutrition a normal deficiency can usually be rectified by eating more fruit and vegetables however those on Diuretics or in a very hot climate may need to take up to 1.5g daily.

Excessive dosages can lead to toxicity in the form of muscular weakness and mental apathy eventually stopping the heart.

Selenium

Selenium is an essential trace element which has recently been classified as one of the most important nutrients necessary for the human body.

One of the major problems in obtaining enough Selenium is that it is absorbed by the plants which we eat from the soil in which it is grown. As most of the soil in the UK is deficient in Selenium, except for the East Anglian area, then it follows that the consumption of home grown produce is going to leave us in most cases short of the ideal intake.

Selenium has been linked to the prevention of cancers, the maintenance of healthy eyes, sight, hair and skin. It has also been shown to be beneficial in the prevention of heart & circulatory problems.

The main sources of natural Selenium are wheat germ, bran, onions, tomatoes, broccoli, tuna fish and kidneys.

There are no specific symptoms of deficiency but as indicated above foods grown in deficient soil or a highly processed diet will both lead to a deficiency.

Dosage

US RDA is 50 -100 mcg
EU RDA is 10 – 75 mcg
Supplement is 50 – 200 mcg

It has been suggested that men should supplement at 75 mcg and women at 60 mcg a day. Doses of up to 1,000 mcg have been used for immune stimulation and anti carcinogenic effects. Selenium can be toxic in very large doses and this reveals itself in the form of blackened fingernails and a garlic odour. Daily doses should not exceed 450 mcg except under the supervision of a qualified healthcare practitioner.

Silicon

Silicon is yet another essential trace element and like so many others its properties are only just beginning to be fully understood.

It is thought that Silicon plays an important part in the formation of human connective tissues, bones, skin and fingernails.

Good natural sources are whole grains, vegetables and seafood. It is also present in hard water areas so there are some benefits to the water that gives us all that limescale.

There are no specific symptoms of deficiency although brittle bones, weakened nails and hair and poor skin condition may all be symptoms.

Dosage

There are no official figures for RDA in either the US or EU although it is thought that we need between 20 & 30 mg per day. Although Silicon is toxic if inhaled there is no evidence of toxicity in food or normal supplementation.

Vanadium

Vanadium is another trace mineral which has only recently been proved to be necessary for human health. Around 1900 it was believed to be a miracle cure by some however unfortunately at the doses that were being prescribed it turned out to be highly toxic and therefore its popularity declined.

It is believed that it may be useful in the control of high blood sugar, may help to prevent tooth decay and encourage normal tissue growth.

Natural sources of Vanadium are seafood.

Once again there are no known symptoms of deficiency however it is thought that diets high in vitamin C may reduce the levels in the body.

There are no RDA figures specified in either the US or EU and there are no supplements which contain just Vanadium although some high end modern multi-vitamin supplements may contain low doses. In high quantities Vanadium is highly toxic and has been linked to manic depression.

Zinc

Zinc is one of the most important trace elements in our diet and it is required for more than 200 enzyme activities within the body.

Zinc is the principal protector of our immune systems and is essential for the structure and function of cell membranes.

It helps prevent blindness due to aging, treats infertility problems, maintains sense of taste and smell, prevents hair loss and treats acne and other skin problems.

Good natural sources of Zinc are meat, mushrooms, oysters, eggs and whole grain products.

Symptoms of deficiency can include the following:
- Poor appetite
- Lethargy
- Abnormal taste, smell & vision
- Slow healing wounds
- Increased susceptibility to infections

Dosage

US RDA is 15mg
EU RDA is 15mg
Supplements 15 – 30mg

The 1988-1991 National Health and Nutrition Examination Survey found that up to 45% of adults over the age of 60 had daily Zinc intakes well below the estimated average requirements.

Supplementation along with a good multi-vitamin is suggested and an increase in Copper and Selenium should be considered. Zinc is thought to not be toxic although doses in excess of 150mg a day may cause nausea and vomiting.

Glucosamine

Once hailed the Holy Grail in the fight against joint pain and arthritis this compound has recently come in for some pretty heavy criticism which suggests that it is a sham and that it has no effect on the human body. So what is the truth after all many of us know people who use Glucosamine and swear by its effectiveness in relieving them from joint pain.

The first thing to consider is where the research against Glucosamine has come from and who has funded it and you will not be surprised to find that it was the people who stand to lose most from its use, the big pharmaceutical companies. After all if people start using Glucosamine and it works they are going to lose out on the profit from their patented anti-inflammatory drugs and the like.

So it's all just a con promoted by the big, bad pharmaceutical companies then! Well if only it was that simple you see there are a few big, bad supplement companies as well and they may not be telling the whole truth either. You see Glucosamine comes in two different types, Glucosamine Hydrochloride (HCL) and Glucosamine Sulphate and because the former has a slightly higher concentration of Glucosamine (83% vs. 80%) it is the one that tends to get used in most of the supplements available today.

But here is the problem it is not the best one to use as it requires the presence of Sulphur to enable it to work and that is why Chondroitin Sulphate is commonly added to the formulae. The problem is that this increases the molecule size to the point where it is difficult for it to be absorbed, in fact up to 70% of the active Glucosamine is wasted.

The solution is to use Glucosamine Sulphate even though it is a far more expensive ingredient and much more difficult to source. You see in tests on people suffering from arthritis and osteoarthritis it has been found that the use of Glucosamine

Sulphate has returned the affected joints to normal function in a very short time. This is due to its almost immediate bioavailability: within 30 minutes of consumption, 87 – 97% is in the blood and within 4 hours it is being absorbed by the joint cells.

So while Glucosamine HCL will not do you any harm it will also not do you as much good as quickly as its more expensive relative Glucosamine Sulphate. Under these circumstances the cheaper version turns out to be more expensive and less effective. So where do the big pharmaceutical companies stand on the use of Glucosamine Sulphate? Well not surprisingly they are silent hoping that you the consumer will think that all Glucosamine is the same and that their drugs are the only true solution to the pain and suffering of joint related disease.

If you suffer from Type II Diabetes then you should speak to your healthcare professional about the effects of Glucosamine as research has indicated that it can worsen Insulin resistance. Otherwise if you suffer from joint pain and want to try a more natural treatment speak to your healthcare professional about the use of Glucosamine but make sure that it is Glucosamine Sulphate that you use as you do not want to waste your money on ineffective treatments.

Coenzyme Q10

Ubiquinone Q10 is a naturally occurring substance and a necessary part of the cells energy metabolism. Without Q10 cells cannot produce the energy that is needed for the multitude of activities that take place inside the body. A cell that lacks Q10 is comparable to an engine without spark plugs.

Much evidence points towards the aging process and several illnesses as factors that deplete the body's supply of and ability to produce Q10. These include problems with the immune system, high blood pressure, excess weight and heart and pulmonary circulation problems. It has also been discovered that some medications such as statins which are used to reduce the cholesterol produced by the liver, by people with heart problems, also have the unwanted side effect of retarding the production of Q10 at the same time.

Research scientists have calculated that a 25% drop in the body's Q10 levels can lead to serious illnesses and that death occurs if the level falls by more than 75%!

The best natural sources of Q10 can be found in meat, eggs, fatty fish, wholemeal products, nuts, broccoli and spinach.

The problem that occurs is that Coenzyme Q occurs naturally in many forms in addition to the Q10 variety which our cells need and our bodies use these other forms by converting them into Q10. It is only through this conversion that our bodies can receive sufficient Q10 and this conversion takes place in the liver. It seems that the liver's ability to carry out this process is weakened first by illness and second by the ageing process. This is an unfortunate situation since many health problems associated with old age, for example fatigue and heart problems, are exactly areas where Q10 has a beneficial effect. In other words, just when the body has most need for Q10 its ability to provide sufficient supplies, regardless of the variety of the diet, begins to regress. It is for this very reason that supplementation is recommended.

There has been no official recommended daily allowance set for Ubiquinone however most experts agree that the daily requirement lies between 10 – 30mg however when treating illness dosages of 100 – 400mg are used. If you are currently taking statins then you should consider taking at least 100mg per day as the statin has the effect of preventing the liver from converting the other forms of Coenzyme Q into Q10.

There has been an important development in the production and use of Q10 in recent years and that has come from the fact that there are actually two forms of Q10 these are Ubiquinone and Ubiquinol. Both forms exist naturally in the human body and in a healthy younger person the ratio is 4:96 and in fact Ubiquinol is actually produced from Ubiquinone in a healthy individual. However in older people or people taking certain medications the body finds it harder to make the conversion if at all. Fairly recently the method of producing the reduced (or active) form of Q10 has been perfected and it is now possible to buy Ubiquinol although the process does make the supplements considerably more expensive. This is somewhat offset by the fact that the Ubiquinol version is believed to be about 8 times more beneficial that the Ubiquinone version.

For anyone interested in learning more about this important substance I would recommend the book 'Q10 Body Fuel The natural way to a healthier body and a longer life' by Dr. Knut. T. Flytlie.

Serrapeptase

You may well not have heard of this substance but it is likely that it will not be too long before it is as well known as aspirin.

Serrapeptase is an enzyme which is fairly new to the scene in that it has only been studied for about 30 years. However in that time it has created quite a stir and the list of conditions which it has been suggested that it can cure has grown so long that if it can only do half of what is claimed it will have earned its title as the 'Miracle' Enzyme. You see Serrapeptase is a Protease Type Enzyme that stops inflammation and dissolves non-vital tissue.

Over the past 30 years studies have indicated that it can benefit in a huge number of conditions including: Arthritis, Inflammatory Migraines/Headaches, and Chest Problems such as Bronchitis, Asthma, Bronchiectasis, Sinus, Blocked Arteries, Fibrocystic Breast Disease, Breast engorgement and Cancers.

Enzymes are catalysts and fulfil many essential functions in the human body. There are Digestive enzymes, Metabolic enzymes and Clean-up enzymes which work with the vitamins and minerals we supply to our bodies and they provide the energy for us to function, the maintenance facilities to repair damaged bodies and the clean up crew to scour out and discard the refuse and waste products and toxins.

On a daily basis we obtain these enzymes from unprocessed, raw or little cooked food or by taking some form of supplementation. Studies have found that a 70 year old has only 20% of the enzymes found in the body of a 20 year old. This is a major part of the cause of age related diseases.

So how many enzymes are there? Well that is difficult to answer, all that we can say is that in 1930 only 80 enzymes had been discovered but by 2000 this had risen to 3,000 enzymes and the figure keeps on rising. In addition in all the studies that have been undertaken there have been no adverse side effects found from the use of enzymes. So if there are no side effects why are doctors not using them? There are many doctors that are starting to use enzymes and other natural supplements but they are a small number who have started to look at medicine from a more eastern viewpoint. Unfortunately in the west our medical culture is more of disease management whereas the eastern culture is more based on health maintenance. In China you pay your doctor when you are healthy not when you are ill so he has a financial interest in keeping you healthy!

Serrapeptase dissolves non-living tissue, blood clots, cysts and arterial plaque and inflammation in all forms. Much of the work on understanding what Serrapeptase can achieve is being undertaken outside the UK in Europe particularly in Germany. There have been some amazing stories about how people who were scheduled for heart bypass surgery were able to come off the surgery list after alternative treatments were tried using Serrapeptase and the previously existing blockages had literally been dissolved away.

The claims for this particular enzyme along with certain other enzymes take up a book on their own and before using these I would recommend that you buy a copy of 'The Miracle Enzyme' by Robert Redfern, you will never think of health care in quite the same way ever again trust me.

Useful Herbs

Detailed below are the 12 most popular herbs along with a quick description of what they are commonly used to treat and when they are best taken for optimum effect:

ALFALFA – is good as an appetite stimulant, tonic, arthritic medicine and cleanser. Works best if taken early in the morning.

BURDOCK – is good as a blood purifier for removing toxins and poisons, liver problems, sores and rashes. It is best taken in the morning and afternoon.

CAPSICUM – is a good digestive aid, a stimulant, aids blood circulation, varicose veins, bleeding and diabetes. It is best taken in the morning and afternoon.

ECHINACEA – is good for helping to remove toxic impurities, blood poisoning, boils, acne and compromised immunity [colds]. It is best taken in the evening.

FENUGREEK – is good for the treatment of tuberculosis, bronchitis, emphysema, sore throat, gout and also acts as a sexual stimulant. There is no known time that is best for using this herb at present.

GARLIC – is good as a digestive aid and in the treatment of congestion, fever, hypertension, intestinal parasites, cancer, immunity, toothache and gangrene. It is best taken between midnight and the early morning.

NETTLE – is good as a digestive aid and in the treatment of breast milk flow, bloody urine, haemorrhoids, excessive menstruation, rheumatism, diarrhoea, grey hair and baldness. It is most effective when taken in the morning and evening.

PEPPERMINT – is good for the relief of nervousness, cramps, coughs, colds, pain, migraines, nausea and stress. It is best taken in the morning and evening.

RED CLOVER – is good for the liver, bladder, relief of constipation, as a digestive aid, a blood purifier and the treatment of leukaemia and other cancers. It is best taken in the early to late morning.

VALERIAN ROOT – is good for spasms, as a sedative, relief of intestinal gas, stomach difficulties, hypertension, migraine headaches, insomnia, cramps, fatigue, nervous breakdown and post traumatic stress. It is best taken in the early morning and late evening.

YARROW – is good for the treatment of spasms, excessive perspiration, intestinal worms, liver problems, blood clots, intestinal gas, gall stones, yeast infection, inflammation and autoimmune disorders. Like Valerian Root it is best taken in the early morning and late evening.

[The above information on common herbs has been taken from 'Rip Off Supplements and how to spot them' by Dr John Heinerman PhD]

Common Ailments

The following information has been taken from the book 'Vitamins & Minerals' by Karen Sullivan.

The following conditions may respond to increased levels of some nutritional elements. This advice in no way replaces that of a physician or health practitioner and before using supplements you should consider seeking expert attention. Never take more than the recommended dose noted on your supplement packaging unless it has been prescribed by a health care professional.

Acne – Try taking a good quality multi vitamin supplement and increase intake of Vitamins E & A and Zinc. Eliminate as much processed food from the diet as possible.

Allergies – Increase your intake of Vitamins B12 & C and try to take a supplement to boost your immune system.

Anaemia – Increase your intake of Iron and Vitamins B1, B6 & C as well as Folic acid.

Arteriosclerosis – Increase your intake of the following vitamins B-complex, A, C & E. Also increase your intake of the minerals Selenium, Magnesium, Manganese and Zinc. Reduce the amount of fats and processed foods in your diet.

Arthritis – Increase your intake of the Vitamins A, B-complex, B5 and D. Also increase your intake of the following minerals, Calcium, Magnesium and Copper.

Asthma – Increase your intake of the vitamins C, A, B2, B5, B6 and E.

Colds – Increase your intake of vitamins C, A & E and minerals Selenium and Zinc.

Cold Sores – Increase your intake of vitamins C, E & B1 along with the mineral Zinc.

Constipation – may respond to an increase in intake of vitamin B-complex and B1. Also increase your daily fibre intake.

Coughs – Increase your intake of vitamins B-complex, C, A & E along with the minerals Selenium and Zinc.

Dandruff – Increase your intake of the vitamins B-complex, C & E and the minerals Selenium and Zinc.

Depression – Increase your intake of vitamins B, C & E together with the minerals Zinc, Magnesium and Calcium.

Diabetes – Increase you intake of the minerals Chromium, Potassium and Zinc and vitamin B-complex.

Diarrhoea – Increase your intake of Potassium along with vitamins B1 & B3. Consume water to flush your system and take a good multivitamin and mineral supplement with food when you are able to eat properly again to replace the lost nutrients.

Eczema – Increase your intake of vitamins A, B-complex, B2, B6, C, E & Biotin and the minerals Zinc & Copper.

Fatigue – Increase your intake of vitamins B6 & B12 and the minerals Calcium, Zinc, Magnesium and if you suspect anaemia Iron.

Glandular Fever – Increase your intake of vitamins B-complex, C, A & E along with the minerals Zinc and Magnesium.

Gout – Increase your intake of Magnesium and vitamins B6 & B12.

Hair Loss – Increase your intake of vitamin B-complex and the minerals Calcium and Magnesium.

Hangover – Take a Vitamin B-complex tablet before you go out drinking, one while you are out and one before retiring to bed. Also take a good multivitamin containing biotin and selenium before going to bed. If you have a hangover when you wake take a multivitamin and mineral tablet twice a day until symptoms cease.

Hay Fever – Increase your intake of vitamin B-complex & C and the minerals Zinc and Selenium.

Headaches – Increase your intake of vitamins B3 & B-complex, in addition increase intake of minerals Calcium and Magnesium.

High Blood Pressure – Increase your intake of the minerals Potassium and Calcium and the vitamins B-complex & E.

Influenza – Increase your intake of the vitamins C, A & B-complex also increase your intake of Zinc.

Insomnia – Take one Calcium and one Magnesium tablet before going to bed and increase your intake of vitamins B3 & B6.

ME – Increase your intake of the vitamins and minerals that boost your immune response including the minerals Selenium and Zinc and the vitamins C, E, B5 & B6.

Menopausal Symptoms - Increase your intake of vitamin E, B6, C, D & B-complex. In addition increase your intake of the minerals Iron and Calcium.

Menstrual Problems – Increase your intake of the vitamins B6, B-complex & B12. Increase your intake of the minerals Iron & Magnesium.

Nausea – Take vitamin B6.

PMS – Increase your intake of vitamin B6, B-complex, B12 & E. Also increase your intake of Magnesium and Calcium.

Psoriasis – Increase your intake of vitamins A, C, E & B-complex. Increase your intake of the mineral Selenium.

Stress – Take a good multivitamin with extra vitamins B-complex, C and E.

Thrush – Increase your intake of the vitamins C, E, A & B-complex. Take additional Selenium and Zinc minerals.

Varicose Veins – Increase your intake of vitamins and minerals which improve circulation which include vitamins C & E and the minerals Boron, Selenium and Silicon.

I hope that the contents of this book have proved both helpful and educational and that as a result you have gained a valuable insight into the world of vitamins and minerals.

As has been reiterated throughout this book you should not self medicate in preference to seeking the assistance of qualified medical and health care professionals.

Hopefully what you have gained by reading this book is an appreciation that there is a valid case for supplementing vitamins and minerals when you are prevented from obtaining them in sufficient quantities from natural sources, or when illness or age prevent you getting them in sufficient quantity.

Until the next time **THANK YOU** for buying this book and I hope that you have gained from the experience of reading it.

Graham Yeomans